Healthy Lifestyle Changes and Weight Reduction Program

Healthy Lifestyle Changes and Weight Reduction Program

Yvan F. Leger

ISBN 978-0-557-48078-4

MESSAGE

Perception is everything in the eyes of the beholder. We live in a world in constant evolution where society demands are brought upon us. To be our best, to look incredible and to convey a sense of achievements . Few can fit that mold and yet we all aspired to reach such incredible heights. What makes a person with similar qualities and educational background achieve wonderful success while the next one with equal affinities barely makes it in life. I believed that the condition of the mind, physically and mentally is the secret to such abundance. You must conditions yourself spiritually and mentally to welcome success. A valuable aspect is to feel healthy and physically fit. This is a key element as your overall positiveness and desire to win will become its driving force. If you' re not healthy or in reasonable shape, all your time will be focus to maintain your overall health conditions. This is a wake up call, for prevention and action. In the next few pages of this program, you will be introduced to a weight reduction program that I hope will be beneficial to you. No need to read a 400 pages diet book and feel exhausted and discourage before you even start. Just a common sense approach to gradually reduce your overall weight and start to feel good about yourself. You will then become more positive, regain energy and become more productive. This in turn will gradually change your life and transform your inner self. So without due hesitation lets plunge into the heart of the matter.

Content

Introduction

Am I to fat, overtired and continuously out of breath. Is my overall health condition improving or deteriorating. Is my reflecting image on peoples interesting or do they find me a nuisance or plain boring. So many questions, and yet so little answers. You have your own personal reason to in bark on this journey, so hopefully you will find your new found avenues within this small booklet. I would like to prone for a minute on the image aspect of the program. I try to put together a solution that will improve your weight, quality of life and overall appearance. This is a key element in order for you to have a most productive and interesting life. If you're always sick, you will lack energy, if you feel unattractive, you will lack motivation and if depress, you will just fall to total desolation. I'm not saying that I have all the solutions to the problems, but I surely have a first step to change the situation. I know that some peoples will tell you that beauty is within but unfortunately, before it is discovered, the exterior must click in action. I'm not inventing the wheel, just a brief reflection on life. Be honest with yourself, our you not more attracted to a person that reflect confidence, charm and good look. I don't know about you, but being a man I surely enjoy looking at a woman that reflect carefulness and sound fashion choices, then one that his always dress in baggy pants with her bra strap hanging down her side. Some peoples have the way of improving their looks and surely conveys confidence. Weight is very important as it gives you that special attractiveness that peoples want to see. Clothes fit's nicer, selection is more subjective and disposition more acute. You feel sure of yourself, and it gives you and add up boost to your self image. Society is imposing directly or indirectly via various medias a sense of standard via the general public. You can have the most pleasant personality, be a great friend but perception is everything to a stranger. Did you ever noticed, in a store or a place that attractive and happy individual seem to have the most attention. I believe this to be normal as they are more pleasant to the view and con way magnetism that we all want to enjoy. Your first contact will indicate a mode that will be perceived by others. They will judge you on physical attractiveness, communication skill and overall energetic chemistry.

Life is sometime not fair, but you should try to arm yourself in emotional skills, physical traits and confidence to confront the situation. Given solutions in this program will definitely help you, but only you are the master of your own determination. You must resolve yourself to totally want the changes and apply effort to achieve them. Sacrifices will be required, but in life nothing is ever made easy. If it was, we would all be attractive, slim, successful and rich. Only few defines changes and take charge, and hopefully you will be the one of the privilege few . Magnetism is key and the program is geared toward accomplishing some of your set goals. The secret is in the presentation, as you must totally change your mental state conditions. Your determination must be your allied or you will fail. One of the most seek resolutions in the New Year is to change our eating habits and become a better and more pleasant person. No one said that it will be done overnight, but little steps can easily leap bond in large and rewarding gains. I know that you want those changes, or you wouldn't have taking the time to acquire this book and read it's content. I was once unsure of myself, overweight and lacking motivation and did procrastinated allot till I decided to take charge and change my life around. I grew to find my physical appearance lacking in many ways. Complexion, body fat, lack of energy and overall demoralized self image. I wanted what the others had, which was motivation, spirit and attractiveness. Not just in the sense of exterior beauty but, a feeling of self worthiness. I stop complaining, threw away some of my old clothes, refresh my look and started this whole brand new program. I gradually cut down on my food intake, changes some of my eating habits and grew more fond of myself after a few short months. There was pain and craving associated with the changes but I was more than ever determine to totally turn my life around. I also read allot, which brought me to put some of my found knowledge into action. I also flirted with lots of magazines, Internet connections and newspapers discussing renewed sense of motivations and self control. I don't want you to become a buff of the information world, but acquiring some references is never a lost cause. Read and you shall master your mind in becoming more intellectual and productive. Rome wasn't built in a day, but small steps made it once, one of the world greatest empire. Remember, you want renewed energy, self motivation and total life new experiences. So this program will start you by reflecting a newer image, self control and sound physical practices. You will develop a new sense of belonging once again to society by a regaining surge of energy. Like someone once said; " Winners are losers, that decided to give it one more try" Good Luck....

Mind Control

Section 2:

This is one of the most important factor of the program. Without it you won't succeed, as you must condition your mind to get ready to accept all changes. You may wish something but it won't happen if you don't apply yourself to it. Sacrifices is a prerequisite, as you will be face with tremendous pressure to fall to temptation. Food is so appealing, restaurants, your old snacks will all be factors that will throw some curves in the beginning. But rest assure that the cause is not totally lost as you will recoup some of your old habits. Naturally it will be in moderations but trust me, that if you follow the program your stomach would have shrunk anyway. I went to the movies the other day and was astonished, at a mid twenty years old gentleman that was eating a popcorn. He had a lovely daughter on his lap, and when I glazed to watch him I noticed that he was consuming to himself a triple large bucket of popcorn. He literately ate the whole amount for the total duration of the movie. No wonder he was about 300 pounds and able to sit on two seats. That proportion of intake is not healthy for you and should be discouraged. If you are that type of person, I strongly suggest that you immediately apply yourself to my program. You may find me critical and harsh, but if I wasn't concern, I surely wouldn't have taken the time to write this book. Eating habits, is the key to survival and longevity. You want to look your best, be physically active and look presentable, and a pot belly, being 300 pounds is surely displeasing to the eye. Especially when you dress up in and old t-shirt and worn off jeans. I'm not here to prejudge people but to show and image that can be surely rejected by society. The greatest of peoples are also subjective to being overweight and emotionally sad. They are your friends, family members and co- workers and should be treated with respect. If they are happy in that conditions, it is their personal choice, but bad eating practice will always results in disease, severe heart conditions and even cancer. I want you to live and enjoy life to it's fullest in the best possible shape and mental state condition. Your mind is the most powerful machinery at your disposal. Maximized its utility and you would see changes that are far exceeding your most imaginable desires. You will control your destiny, your appearance and even your projection on society. You are the student, that will one day grow to be the master. You will take your life from the gutter and scoop it into dream realities that you have never imagined. Your effort and sheer determination, will be predispose you to a life of renewed energy. The challenges ahead of you, will only be beneficial if you apply yourself to the solution. It is vital that you keep focus in order to fully enhance the main principles. You will have to conditions yourself to tough time ahead but still maintain your determination. Affirmations and visualizing your goals will be your main weapon. There is no coming back, or you will fail. The results will only be reflected by the effort that you will put into it. But rest assure that if you're persistent and consistent, changes will occur. It may take a few months to a year to achieved, but persistence will be the driving force of your desired goal. Now since we are talking about mind control, I would like to stress the importance of acquiring new found and renewed knowledge. I'm not trying to be a geek or a dysfunctional intellectual, but knowledge is key in a positive approach. Did you ever had a dream of becoming a writer, a carpenter, a programmer or even a designer. The choices are countless and the opportunity without end. Your desired goals, is only a finger tip away from your life. Some little girls, plays with dolls and eventually become designers, some boys plays with trucks and eventually become truckers. Whatever you wish for, can be achieved regardless of your age, physical condition or financial desperation. Victor Hugo, wrote some of his greatest masterpiece after the age of 60. The author of the Harry Potter saga wrote her novel in the corner of a restaurant in order to keep warm. There is no reason for you not to attained your goals, if you truly desire them. Motivation and mind control are the most crucial elements required in order to master your new found energy. But like only so few of us, only a small proportion of individuals with apply the science. There also an indicating source that dictate, that whenever you read and acquire knowledge your wealth is eventually increased in proportion. I'm not talking going to University and get a degree, but to simply apply the art of reading. You become versatile in conversational abilities, become more aware of your surroundings and have a more openness toward the world. Your eyes are no longer shut, and you can easily find the goodness in everyone you meet. Sure there will still be some distasteful peoples around to cause you some problems, but at least you wouldn't be one of them. But later on in the program, I will discuss various approach to developing a more positive attitude. It's not an easy process as you must rewired your brain wave to accept changes, but there a few methods that can path the way to a brighter future. But without due hesitation, let's go to the actual step of my technique.

Equipment

Section 3:

The only devices that would be required is a weight scale, a note pad and maybe a calorie intake book. But I have included within this package a listing of calorie choice products for your own consumption.

Beginning

Section 4:

Now that you have set yourself to improving your overall image and health conditions the following steps would prove to be necessary. Your age is totally irrelevant, but your mental state condition is prevalent. This will dictate your willingness to change and acceptance of yourself as a vital member of society. In other word, you must reflect a positive attitude, before you undergo this program. Negative concept does not lead to success, only sheer determination of accomplishment. You will see that throughout your journey, I will always try to reinforced your self confidence.

On a piece of paper, highlight in large bold letters the word{DISCIPLINE}, as a reminder of your self consciousness. Before you start your day in the morning, go through your set goals within your mind. This will condition your body and mind to slowly accept all changes that it will endure. One your paper, you will have incorporated brief sentences of your set goals as a reminder.

Examples:

> I want to be slimmer .
>
> I want to feel good about myself
>
> I want a better image
>
> I want to be attractive

There is countless reason for changes, but gear them positively toward your own references. Another one could be to age gracefully or improve my overall health conditions. Your goals, your desires so you be the judge and take charge.

Afterward you will mark on the same piece of paper, your deficiencies such as large belly, skin condition, tiredness and naturally your excess weight. This is very important as everything will be centered around it.

On another paper mark the date and your current weight. This will serve as a starting point, so be accurate. Every seven days afterward you will add the date followed by your current weight. This will act as a guideline to evaluate your overall progression. At first your weight reduction will be moderate to acceptable with increment progression. Since your body will be slowly reprogramming itself, don't fall to discouragement. At first you may have some relapses, due to hunger but just keep plugging at it. Relapses at first will occur, but just motivated yourself by going over your goals. As you become more conscious of the changes your body and stomach will become less dependent on food. This is because your stomach would have shrunk, and dependency on food will be less.

After a few weeks, a new phenomena will surface within your dieting routine. Suddenly the loss of weight will start to stagnate. All thought you are controlling your eating habit and eating more moderately, your weight loss will be limited. What you will have to do is to jolt your stomach by going and having a good eating frenzy. A large supper or an entire barrel of popcorn at the movies. What is occurring is that your metabolism, has accepted your new found eating habits and went into a slow mode. It need less intake, and has reprogramed itself to survive on less. By jolting your metabolism, you will quick start it again.

During those phases, you will naturally fall to hunger as your stomach will be indicating to you that you must eat more in order to survive. Temptation will be great so I suggest that you try to exercise your mind to other projects. A hobby or an active mind controlling board game. Not a passive one or your mind will just be thinking of satisfying it's craving. Video or board games are quite suitable as you must constantly keep focus on the play. Drink plenty of water, and maybe go to bed earlier during the first few weeks of the program.

Spacing

Section 5:

I want to stress out that this is not a race, and should be taken as a gradual phase. Changes and weight reduction will definitely occur within your own body composition. There are billions of peoples on this nice planet of ours and everyone is different, but rest assure results will happen. Don't try to change yourself overnight, and also if in doubt please contact you physician. Factors that are important to consider, is your overall health conditions. If you have glands problem, then you should contact your doctor, before you apply my theory.

I also strongly discourage fasting days. Unless for religious purpose, they can be quite harmful to your body then beneficial. They put an overall stress on the metabolism and created a panicking sense of craving that can be disastrous. You would want to indulged yourself and would easily fall prey to temptation. Every justifications in your mind would become acceptable to engage into an eating frenzy. Remember this should only be use as a measure to counter act slow metabolism process and not to justify hunger.

Also you should refrain from purchasing snacks and high calorie food. Buy healthy food and store away in your cupboard those restaurant coupons that serve as an incentive. Don't worry you will have a chance to use them later on within the course of this program.

The secret in spacing is to slowly regain control of your eating habits. You can't put an overdue stress on yourself but you will have to slowly diminish your intake. Your body will then gradually adjust to those changing all thought it will try to test your resolve. It's not going to be an easy process, but you're looking for a long term solution. If you keep committed to your goals success will follow.

Exercising

Section 6:

Certain form of exercise can be quite beneficial to you, if taken in moderation. I'm not a heavy buff of exercising but do enjoy swimming and walking. I'm aware of the beneficial attributes offered by a gym but not everyone is totally inclined to actually enjoy them. Seniors or severe obese peoples may feel intimidated by the younger or more slim individuals. They could easily feel pressured or discouraged by their surroundings. All thought it can be a vital a source of calorie reductions, the membership in itself can be very expensive.

A source of advice to new beginners would be to slowly undertake moderate exercise, followed by a convenient sport activity and gradually work toward a gym fitness program if they wish.

I'm not an gym activity person myself so I would like to suggest to peoples with similar traits to undertake a 30 minutes routine walk every day. It's probably one of the best form of exercise that is easily accessible to everyone. Cross country in the winter is also great, but I strongly discourage jogging as it put an overdue stress on the heals.

Another form of valuable and beneficial exercise is swimming. Your whole body is set in motion and you definitely feel rejuvenated after a water session. For the ladies who feel shy about their bodies, I recommend the one piece bathing suit. They come in all style and forms, for young and old. The idea is to enjoy yourself and feel good mentally and physically. Encourage yourself through visualization of your body being transform and a sense of renewed energy would slowly emerged. If new at it, just take your time and you will gradually regain a set motion.

Cycling is also a most encouraged form of exercise and can be quite rewarding when cruising sight seeing area.

Food Intake

Section 7:

This is a very important part of the program and directives should be followed carefully. Remember the saying that said."You are what you eat" You may feel discouraged by the terminology, but if you do eat like a (pig) then don't be surprise by the results. You will expand your body, built fat and simultaneously deteriorate your entire body. It will show poor skin complexion, heavy body mass and sign of fatigue. The solution is to take charge, confront the situation and undertake a plan of action to improve your overall health and image.

Intake is very important to weight reductions and must be controlled carefully. You don't want to do excess or fall below a respectable form of calories count tolerance. Your body needs to feed itself but the amount will determine the weight loss that will result.

I prefer the moderation aspect to a strenuous accelerated plan. You may have been in your conditions for many years, so don't push yourself to the limit. For the younger ones, the issue would be to regain self confidence via a well balance and healthy regime.

Now I would like to bring to your attention that in order to burn one pound of fat you must burn 3500 calories. This can be done by a moderate to heavy form of exercise plan and sound eating practice. You be the judge and preset your plan. But remember you cannot go lower than 1000 calories a day as it is the threshold to survival. Some experts recommend a daily doze to be set of at 1250 calories for women and 1800 calories for men.

And interesting avenue to health conscious peoples would be to compare products label for calories and beneficial properties. I was overwhelmingly surprised when I was able to substitute similar eating products with more competitive and healthy choices. A comparison was various soups pack with sodium and increasing large amounts of calories. Shopping within the same grocery store I was able to find similar products with excellent taste and less calories.

Be the judge and go in a grocery store establishment of your choice and have fun with a piece of paper. Substitute all your bad food habits choices for more healthy and nutritional comparison value.

Then go home and slowly start to change your cupboard with your new found resource. Try to prevent yourself from buying snacks food, as you may easily fall to temptation if they are readily available. Reserve some of those products as a reward on the weekend via a restaurant or movie.

The aspect of the program is to gradually control your eating habits, to an eventually more moderate food intake. You will sustain your weight via sound eating practices. You will change the format of your meal via a more slowly integrated vegetables and fruits diet. This will increase your energy, make you more slimmer and by all mean more healthier. Body fat would diminish and be more so, as time goes by. Your skin would become healthier, as you would have incorporated a balanced diet comprise of fruits. A listing of fruits and its attributes are listed in the next few pages. You will see that a combination of various berries will prove to be increasingly beneficial.(blueberries, raspberries, strawberries etc...). A suggested reading or research on the Mediterranean diet is strongly recommended.

Another important aspect is not to drastically cut your food intake to the point of starvation. Overdue stress on the body is not recommended, especially at the beginning of the program. The solution reside in controlling the calories intake. But do try to eliminate the consumption of chips, chocolate bars and candies. They are full of calories including drinking pop sodas. But a valuable source of chocolate that is favored for therapeutic value is cacao. Accordingly to my research cacao has beneficial value such as cutting cancer, increase magnesium helping blood flow and improving skin complexion. I recommended two small cubes of a 75% cacao chocolate bars to be sufficient as a daily dosage. Do not eat the whole chocolate bars as it would add up considerably in calories intake. For the braver of us you could even attempt to increase it to an 85% cacao bar.

Limitation is also a key element to the program. Diminish your bad habits by converting them into positive choices. If you currently drink three cans of soft drink a day like I use to do, try to reduce it to only one can a day. If you took cake in the morning, afternoon and night, then try a muffin for breakfast or diner and a piece of cake for supper.

Just use sound judgment and common sense to adjust it to your particular circumstances. The whole concept is to prevail in reducing calories intake to a more acceptable level. For recap purposes, you will combine a more moderate exercise program with a more balance and healthy choices diet. Sacrifices will be needed as you must changes sometimes years of bad habits, but replacing your snacks with fruits choices that you like would gradually ease the craving pains. And naturally drinking plenty of water is always recommended.

Remember eating all sort of fatty foods is a detriment to your body, so try to look for lean meats when shopping. Turkey is also a recommended choice, but try to stay clear of process meat. Also like I said earlier, try to substitutes similar choices and taste with more highly recommended package.(read the label content)

After a few months you will notice that you will feel more energized, healthy and in control of yourself. Your body would have adjusted to its new regime and you will feel more rejuvenated by your new found appearance. You will shine physically and emotionally.

But before we leave this step of the program, there is some key elements that you should be aware of. Negative points that can be damaging to the body is related through alcohol and cigarettes consumption. Excessive alcohol intake can be damaging to the liver and weaken the immune system. It should be taken in moderation as drinking binge definitely increase your calories intake by an urge to indulged yourself with fatty food afterward. A recommended suggestion, would be limit alcohol consumption to a mere social activity. I'm aware that for some individuals, it is a valuable source of satisfaction, so eliminating would be out of the question. What I may say, is just to have it in moderation, and try to eliminate the surge to eat afterward in order to reduce the due stress on the body.

One element that I could find no value into it and highly cancerous was cigarettes. Unfortunately you will have to try to eliminate that addiction because no beneficial value could be extracted from it. Except for calming nerves when in panic it only adds deterioration to vital organs of the body. There are frightening facts associated with this sort of addictions. For drug users, my only suggestions is to seek help by recommended agencies in your area as these addictions is the more severe of them all. These suggestions could also apply for alcoholism and heavy smokers. The positive part of rehab is many of these programs are sponsored by various health organization. If in doubt just consult various listings within the Internet, or for alcohol related issues just join alcoholic anonymous.

The importance issues to food intake is to be aware that there is conditional circumstances that brings your body under due pressure. You will have to master those conditions in order to feel more in control of yourself and gradually overturn the deteriorating process of aging. You have to look at it as a long term goal in order to increase your longevity and self awareness. All age group can benefit from the program, by improving overall heath conditions. Again I would like to stress that if you have heavily medical conditions prior to this program you should consult your physician if in doubt. The reason I would like to stress this point , is that no one in poor health conditions should conduct any sort of diet need changes without due approval. This program, like any others in the industry, are usually related to average folks with average conditions and open disposition to changes.

Before leaving this final aspect, I would like to highlight some of the beneficial value once again.

a- Improved energy

b- Sustained health changes

c- better skin complexion

d- elimination of bad toxic

e- weight control

f- improved self image

There could be countless of other features but the overall sense of value can be concurred in the selections above. Before we past to another step let me totally congratulated you in assimilating this portion of the program so far. I want to reinforced your desire to changes as potential value to a more healthy body is key to a more satisfying life. Don't forget your goals that were highlighted at the beginning of this undertaking as they are key to your success. They are attainable and visualization of your end results and should serve as a boost to its accomplishment. If not sure of the philosophy, reread the first few portions and draw out its main points on a piece of paper as a reference. For a bonus supplements I have included the next few pages pertaining to the benefits of fruits and vegetables.

ANNEX

Fruits:

Berries group(probably one of the most beneficial to your body)

Blackberries:

> Strong antioxidant full of vitamins A and C.
> Helps to eliminate cholesterol.
> Prevents several types of infections and cancers.
> Help against diabetes.
> Prevent some age-related cognitive degenerations.

Blueberries:

> Strong antioxidant enhance with vitamins C and E.
> Protect the body against long term and damaging effect associated with aging.
> Promote urinary tract health.
> Good on blood vessels and the treatment of varicose veins.
> Increase motor behavioral learning abilities and memory.

Raspberries

> Help to prevent cancers.
> Stop the growth of potential harmful form of cancers.
> • Ideal fruit for dieting as its properties helps to increase metabolism, resulting in burning fat. *

Strawberries

> Excellent source of vitamin A, C. E and K.
> Vitamin K is and element needed in preventing hemorrhage, or excessive loss
> of blood in an accident.
> Full of folate, thiamin, riboflavin, and Omega-3.
> Excellent antioxidant.
> Enhance memory function capability.
> Keep bad cholesterol away that could cause damage to the artery walls.
> Helps against anemia and fatigue.

Apples:

> Reduce skin diseases, arthritis and asthma.
> Excellent against insomnia and Gallbladder stones.
> 2 apples a day can lower your cholesterol by 10%.

Apricots:

> Full of beta carotene which helps in combating infections.
> Excellent agent against skin problems.(pimples and skin disorder)
> Help against asthma, bronchitis and toxemia.
> Bananas:
> Rich in vitamins B6 and folic acid.
> Good against high cholesterol and cramps associated with PMS.
> Excellent agent against intestinal disorders and ulcers.
> Help in constipation and diarrhea relief.

Cantaloupe:

> Promote lung health and vision.
> Important in production of new cells during pregnancy.
> Helps against fever, skin diseases and arthritis.
> Reduce constipation and high blood pressure.

Cherries:

> Excellent source of potassium, magnesium and calcium.
> Full of vitamins B6,C,K, thiamin and riboflavin.
> Reduce pain due to arthritis, gout and headaches.
> Contain melatonin which help in boosting the immune system.
> Reduce the risk of heart attack and cancer.

Cranberries:

> The juice is excellent against cystitis and urinary infections.
> Immune system booster.
> Provide relief to asthma patient.
> Help against the development of kidney stones.

Dates:

> Beneficial against anemia, constipation and fatigue.
> Good against preventing abdominal cancer.
> Helps to improve sex stamina and sterility.
> Remedy against alcohol intoxication.(drink water with dates)

Grapefruit:

> Protect against infections and cancer.
> Excellent antioxidant food.
> Excellent in weight reductions at it is full of fat burning enzymes.
> Help reduct the risk of heart disease.
> Helped repair damage (DNA) in human prostate cancer cells.

Grapes:

> Good blood and body builder.
> Help to reduce harmful blood clot.
> Ideal for cleansing and detoxing the body.
> Help to protect the heart and reduce cancer.

Kiwi:

> Full of vitamin C.
> Good for digestion and the immune system.
> Help to maintain the heart and reduce blood pressure.
> Help against respiratory health issues such as wheezing, shortness of breath and high coughing.
> Antioxidant and rich in enzymes.

Lemons:

> Rich in vitamin C, calcium, iron and magnesium.
> Protect against infection and cancer.
> Effective gargle(diluted half in half with hot water) against ulcers and sore throats.
> Natural antiseptic when the juice is applied on cuts and infection areas.
> Help in preventing diabetes.
> Relieve a toothache when fresh juice is applied on the area.
> Lemon is a blood purifier and eliminator of toxins.

Mango's:

> Good for immune system.
> Help protect against cancer.
> Effective in relieving clogged pores of the skin.
> Help against acidity and digestion.

Orange:

Effective during cough, cold and fevers.
Ideal against constipation, scurvy and headache.
Lowers blood pressure and cures vomiting.
Prevents kidney stone and asthma.
Helps in rheumatism, hypertension, sun and heat stroke.

Special note: Orange juice may help some alcoholics in cutting the urge to drink.

Papaya:

Helps in digestion.
Prevents constipation and nausea.

Pears:

Full of Vitamin A, B2, C and iron.
Helps to lower cholesterol.
Best and safer fruit for infants.
Beneficial to colon health when eaten in its natural state.
Helps in inflammation and is an immune booster.

Peach:

Extreme high vitamin A content
Helps against the inflammation of the stomach(Gastritis) and kidneys
Relieves constipation, bronchitis and asthma.
And aid to removing worms from intestinal tract.
Beneficial to skin and color complexion.

Pineapple:

A cancer protector fruit.
Good for cold and to loosen mucus.
Effective for bones growth in young peoples and strengthen bones in older individuals.

Plums:

Positive source of potassium, Vitamin A and E.
Stimulate blood circulation and healthy tissues' growth.

Watermelon:

> Helps against colon and prostate cancer.
> Highest concentration of lycopene.
> Is an antioxidant fill with Vitamins A and C.

VEGETABLES

Asparagus:

> Helps in the treatment of rheumatism and arthritis.
> Helpful with women around their menstrual cycle.

Avocado:

> Beneficial to ulcer patients.
> Good for women in their menopause.
> Helps against constipation.

Bean Sprouts:

> Very good against cancer and fatigue.
> And immune system booster.
> Good source of vitamin C and low in calories.
> Beets:
> A vital source for a healthy metabolism.

Broccoli:

> High antioxidant with property agents in reducing cancer.
> Effective against lung, stomach and colon cancer.
> Rich in vitamins beta-carotene, C and E.
> Effective against bacteria that causes peptic ulcers.

Brussels sprouts:

> Strong agent against lung and colon cancer.
> Rich in vitamin C and low in fat and calories.

Cabbage:

> Perfect against anemia and pregnant women.
> A cancer reducer especially lung.
> Full of vitamin C and iron.

Carrots:

> May have an ability to reverse the symptoms of cancer.
> Beneficial for the eyes, skin and lungs.
> Improves the heart and circulation system.
> An energetic liver booster.
> Full of vitamin A carotenes, K and Biotin.
> And agent against cardiovascular disease and cancer.
> Eating one carrot a day could reduce lung cancer by 50%.
> Excellent ingredient against post menopausal breasts cancer.
> Protection against the development of cataracts.
> Beta Carotene that prevents cell degenerations and the aging process.

Note; Some research has determined that since carrots is a nerve tonic, it should not be taken during a pregnancy. It may induce abortion.

Cauliflower:

> General immunity protecting cancer agent.
> Contain indole-3-carbinol that affect the metabolism of estrogen.
> A preventer agent against breast and female related cancers.

Corn:

> High in nutrients and fibers.
> Positive in the generation of new cells.
> Full of vitamin C which is a diseases fighter.
> Beneficial to women prior and during pregnancy.
> Helps to lower cholesterols levels.
> Reduce blood sugar levels in diabetics. (fiber)

Cucumbers:

> Helpful agent in stomach and chest problems, arthritis and gout.
> The high sulfur content help in the growth of hair.
> Helps to prevent the splitting of nails(fingers/toes)
> Cucumber juice also helps in the teeth and gums diseases.
> The vegetable is also ideal to improve the texture of your skin.

Garlic:

> Contains allicin with help to reduce unhealthy fats and cholesterol.
> An antioxidant that helps to reduce blood clotting.
> An anti-cancer agent and immune system booster.
> Good for the heart, hair and cough.

Lettuce:

> The only attributes is that it is low in calories.

Mushrooms:

> Full of nutrients and vitamin B12
> Rich in potassium, phosphorous and low in calories.
> Helps to reduce blood pressure and strokes.
> Has positive effect on gall bladders.

Onions:

> Low in calories with vitamins B and C.
> Beneficial in reducing blood clotting and raise healthy cholesterols
> Effective against Salmonella and E. coli.
> Positive in treating coughs, colds, asthma and bronchitis.
> Helps against reducing tumors in the colon.
> Recognized as a beneficial value by the World Health Organization.

Green Peppers:

> A protector against cancer and heart disease.
> Helps against liver disease, obesity, constipation and arthritis.

Red Peppers:

> Full of vitamins A. C, K, B6 and capsaicin(natural pain killer).
> A protector against age-related eye problems.
> An agent preventer against prostate cancer, and cancer of the bladder, cervix and pancreas.

Yellow Peppers:

A protector against cancer and heart disease.

Potatoes:

Excellent for weight loss diets.(slow down digestion.)
High in carbohydrates, vitamins B, C, potassium and fiber.

Note: Green bits on the skin are poisonous and should be removed.

Spinach:

Full of beta-carotene, carotenoids lutein and zeaxanthin.
Helps against age-related macular degeneration(AMD)and eye disease.

A transporter of calcium which help to reduce osteoporosis.
An agent against Crohn's disease.

Tomatoes: (may also be classified as a fruit)

Low in sodium helping to fight against high blood pressure.
Beneficial against cancers(cells) and heart disease.
Large amount may improve skin texture and color.
Excellent blood purifier and beneficial against preventing hemorrhage.
Protects the liver against cirrhosis and hear disease.

Turnips:

Excellent source of vitamin B6, C, E, fiber, calcium and copper.

Zucchini:

Ideal for diets as it is very low in calories.
Helping agent against scurvy and bruising.
Supports the arrangement of capillaries.
Help in preventing multiple sclerosis(MS)

Miscellaneous Elements

Fish:

> Great source of Omega-3 fatty acids that promotes healthy heart and brain.
> Also reduce blood pressure and prevents arthritis.

Green Tea:

> Helpful in the prevention of cancer, high cholesterol levels and infections.
> Good against rheumatoid arthritis and coronary artery disease.

Olive oil:

> Protection against heart disease.
> Beneficial against ulcers and gastritis.
> Lower blood pressure and reduce the risk of Alzheimer and Gallstones.

Nuts:

> Helps to reduce sudden cardiac death.
> Full of protein, fiber, Vitamin E and selenium.

I hope that this short list of healthy products would prove to be beneficial in your quest for a better health. All thought they are in point form, it gives you an overall picture of what is out there for your personal consumption. Not all products are listed, but I wanted to give you a brief list of what is available out there.

Now that we have completed this portion of the program let's leap forward to brief examples, gathered within my own personal journey to health improvement.

Examples

Section 8:

Within my own technique, I was able to reduced my weight by 20 pounds in about 18th weeks. Now you will tell me that some of those expensive programs can give you up to 7 pounds weight reductions per week. But I fear it is mere illusion or damaging to your health. They can promise you the world, but it doesn't mean that they can deliver it. All bodies are different, but a more sound and balanced diet is always preferred in my book then a hastily fast approach. You want your metabolism to accept the changes and not give it a radical shock.

The idea in my mind is to trigger a new mental philosophy to your body and to slowly shift toward a new and rewarding approach. I strive for a longer solution and not a monthly paid subscription to a clinic. I also invite you to diversify your course meal, by researching or browsing through recipes books at your local library. Diversity is the key, as we sometimes seem to be trending on the same kind of foods. That trend can bore us in our eating habits and we easily resolve ourselves to restaurants. The world is so rich with cultures and culinary innovation that we should all lean toward learning new its benefits.

A good example is the Mediterranean cuisine which is probably one of the best source of healthiest and nourishing products. The objectives are to replace some old habits with new and positive and more productive choices. You must stimulate changes and be in full compliance with yourself. Success will only derived from a most determine and highly motivated individual. But before we leave this portion of the program lets recap some of the studied points that we are now undertaking.

A- Try to eliminate one bad habit a week. Like reducing the intake of pop sodas.

B- Introduce various portions of vegetables and fruits in your daily routine.

C- Buy smaller plates and cover it with your desired portion of a meal. Many establishments in Europe has reduced their plates only to serve the appropriated amount of food required. In North America we have the tendency of overfilling our plates with enormous amount of food that eventually ended up into waste baskets. We also overfill ourselves resulting in heart burn or accelerated rate of weight growth.

D- Try to introduce small breaks during your daily routine in order to snack on a fruit or some vegetables. It will cut down on some of your food cravings prior to a lunch or supper.

E- Drink plenty of water, as it helps to reduce the surge of food attack and it cleanse your body.

F- Gradually reduce your eating habits with healthy one, but only with products that you feel comfortable with.

G- Discovery is the key, so try to find new recipes that you would enjoy within a positive nutritional value and acceptable calories.

H- As the week progress, your stomach will shrink and the needs for foods will become easily controllable.

Before we leave this section, you must understand that we are trying to achieve a sound and balance approach. No one is asking you to go and ran a marathon, or to starve yourself to death, but merely to be consistent. You must first take small steps and eventually the gain would result in larger steps for the future. You must be moving in synchronization with your body. You must evaluate your situation and constantly keep in mind your desires and set goals.

Another aspect is to consciously start to feel good about yourself. You have set a mission and you are now pursuing that plan. Later on I will discuss positiveness and renewed energy. It is vital, as your state of mind depends on it for survival. It is quite and art to be positive, but unfortunately many of us are more driven by negativism.

In the following list I have added various supplements to be review by you, depending of your preferences. Also here is a summary list of weight requirements for your gender and height.

Female 4' 10" to 5 feet= 115 to 120 lbs
5' 1" to 5' 3"= 122 to 128 lbs
5' 4" to 5' 6"= 133 to 140 lbs
5' 7" to 5' 9"= 143 to 150 lbs
5' 10" to 6 feet= 153 to 159 lbs

Men 5' 1" to 5' 3"= 134 to 139 lbs
5' 4" to 5' 6"= 142 to 148 lbs
5' 7" to 5' 9"= 151 to 157 lbs
5' 10" to 6 feet= 160 to 167 lbs
6' 1" to 6' 3"= 171 to 179 lbs

This is an average standard chart of measurement but body frames may slightly change some of the weight requirements.

Body Fat: Acceptable body fat as recommended by the American Council on Exercise.

Female: Essential fat: 10-12%
Athletes: 14-20%
Fitness: 21-24%
Acceptable 25-31%
Overweight 32-41%
Obese 42% +

Men Essential fat 2-4%

Athletes 6-13%
Fitness 14-17%
Acceptable 18-26%
Overweight 27-37%
Obese 38% +

The ratios for women is higher due to childbearing and hormonal functions.

Blood Pressure

Blood pressure chart accordingly to age.

Systollic Range	Age	Min	Average	Max
	15-19	105	117	120
	20-24	108	120	132
	25-29	109	121	133
	30-34	110	122	134
	35-39	111	123	135
	40-44	112	125	137
	45-49	115	127	139
	50-54	116	129	142
	55-59	118	131	144
	60-64	121	134	147

Diastolic Range	Age	Min	Average	Max
	15	73	77	81
	20	75	79	83
	25	76	80	84
	30	77	81	85
	35	78	82	86
	40	79	83	87
	45	80	84	88
	50	81	85	89
	55	82	86	90
	60	83	87	91

Supplements

Section 9:

Many of us have tendencies to take vitamins or supplements, to enhance our quality of life. So in the next few pages I have driven an abbreviated list of vitamins and supplements to serve as a guideline. I only listed the most popular one along with its merit. It is written in point form, so not all benefits are listed. For additional information please contact various resource material or research on the Internet.

Vitamin A:(Beta carotene)

Important element to improving your eyes night vision.
Enhance immunity system and growth.
– Helps to built stronger bones.
– Helps against cancer and various disease.
– An agent against heart disease and stroke.
– Lowers blood cholesterol
*** Very positive in woman wanted to improve skin condition and slowly reduce the aging process. Also beneficial to children with respiratory problems.

Source of Beta carotene is: carrots, apricots, pumpkin, spinach, cantaloupe, sweet potato and broccoli.

B1(Thiamin)

– Converts blood sugar into energy.
– Good for nervous system.
– Excellent for cardiovascular and muscular function.

Found in pork, whole grain cereals, whole wheat flour and kidney beans.

B2:

Helps in red cell growth.
Promotes healthy skin and good vision.

Found in enriched bread and cereals, dairy products and green leafy vegetables.

B3:

Helps the digestive system.
Helps healthy skin and nerves.

Found in poultry, fish and peanuts.

B5:

A beneficial factor for the break down of carbohydrates in the body.

Found in peas and yellow beans, poultry, fish and whole grain cereals.

B6:

Help brain function
Help the body into converting protein into energy.
Prevent skin diseases.

Found in poultry, pork, fish, eggs, soybeans, whole grains and bananas.

B9:

Help maintain the flow of new cells and promote production of new ones.
Help to prevent anemia.

Found in Broccoli, asparagus, mushrooms, liver, dry beans and peas.

B12:

Promote a healthy nervous system.
Help to increase white cells and the maturation of red cells.

Found in meats, chicken, fish, milk products, eggs and cheese.

C:

Helps in healing wounds.
Promote healthy gums and teeth.
Strengthen immune system.

Found in citrus juices, fruits(orange etc...), tomatoes, berries, green and red pepper, broccoli ans spinach.

D:

Help bones and tooth formation.
Agent against osteoporosis.
Supports muscle and nervous system.
Keeps a balance within bone and blood calcium.

Found in fortified milk, eggs, tuna and cereals.
This element can also be acquired by sun exposure.

E:

Powerful antioxidant.
Promote a healthy circulatory system.
Increase wound healing.
Prevents sterility and muscular dystrophy.

Found in avocado, whole grain products, nuts, liver and peanut butter.

F:

Excellent in kidney function and bone growth.
Necessary element for blood clotting(stops the bleeding)

Found in spinach, beef liver, green tea and cheese

These are just a small sample selections of various vitamins, but a wide selection is readily available within your favorite pharmacy or super market. You should also consider Omega-3 supplement for a daily dosage for your body.

I would also like to stress that there are various needs depending of each individual pref rence, so just be synchronization with your body. You personally no your needs and deficiencies, so try to correct the weakness if desired by a supplement.

Self Image

I would like to stress the importance of being positive toward your goal and reflect on your image. You must be in full control of your desired goals, as it is a key element to your success. Visualization is the tools to achieved your set results and you must constantly remind yourself of the reward attached to your achievements. Before going to bed you should condition your sub conscious mind to accept your objectives through repetition.

Self image is also not just related to weight, but to a philosophy. The way you address people, the way you interact with your neighbor, are all factors that will define you. Your disposition toward a friend, colleague or an acquaintance is the source by where peoples will judge you. The first impression is very important, as it may seal your faith toward a new found stranger. This is due to the fact that in absence of knowledge, we would easily judge someone on their appearance, facial expression(smiling etc...) or voice tone. Don't be perplex, as it is a natural human phenomena that mostly all of us engaged ourselves in. We pre-judge peoples without facts or personal characteristics.

When you are totally sure of yourself , you will definitely attract positive attributes in your life. Remember, everyone want to be with a winner, so work toward defining your self worth and improving your image. Here are a few steps to achieved those desired goals.

A: Constantly remind yourself of your worthiness in life.

B: Boost your self image by eating properly and reducing your weight to

acceptable levels.

C: Change your wardrobe, if you feel that you have overdone your clothes existence. You may be surprise, how a new dress, or a suit can bring about renewed personal changes. You feel excited and entice to show your new clothes to someone near you.

D: Stop finding excuses for yourself within your poor performance behavior. You are in charge of your destiny and only you can change it's direction. In other word, get rid of self pity. In order to be a winner, you must think like a winner.

E: Keep yourself active, mentally and physically. A walk, swimming, skiing etc... and also reading and playing community activities(games etc...) I would also like to point out the importance of reading, as it is a self image booster. More knowledgeable you become on various topics and more versatile you become in engaging a conversation and be more appreciative by your surroundings. An open minded person, is more likely to be welcome by their peers, then a close and narrow minded individual.

F: Pamper yourself. Go to a movie with a friend, buy yourself something that you long desired, or mainly enrolled yourself into a hobby. Examples; Pottery, sewing, woodworking, collecting, antiques etc... The opportunity is endless. You may even consider doing volunteer work, such as helping the poor s. the orphans, your local hospital or even helping adults to learn to read.

Overall there are countless measures to achieve positiveness, so just draw on

your mental ability, and the door shall open.

Interrelation skill may have to be develop, especially among shy individuals, but little step are far better then no step at all. You may merely say hi, or even open a door to a stranger, but those are steps that would eventually give you assurance in the long run. No need for long conversation, just an acknowledgment. Eventually you will be able to approach more easily a co-worker or even a total stranger in a coffee shop.

The picture that I'm trying to draw to your attention, is a condition in which you feel comfortable with yourself and willing to open yourself to satisfying relationship.

Taking care of yourself, physically, emotionally, and spiritually is a complement to your self image. If you take care of yourself, body and soul your counterpart may just noticed those changes and feel more attracted to you, or have a desire to change themselves.

You will also be valued by your peers. which in turn will make you feel more confident and self assure. Also remember to try to reflect your personality that you wish to project within your attire. Stay away from ragged clothes, as it's make peoples look like losers , out of style and uneducated. You may find me hard, but society does reflect such sentiments. Wear those type of clothes within your indoor surroundings.

Another aspect which is as equally important is hygiene. This would apply to both gender and is not merely restricted to women. A man should be properly groom and shave in order to reflect neatness. A woman should display a certain sense of disposition, within her hair and overall looks.

You may also wish to improve your facial skin complexion(men or women) by using a gentle facial scrub product or moisturizing cream. These products are easily available for both genders in your appropriated pharmacy or super store. You're eating habits will also add to your complexion renewed look, and bring changes within your body.

Take the time to explore those avenues and countless doors will open for you in the future. Positiveness always attract beneficial values. In order to achieve a worthwhile and valuable change in your life, you will have to take a risk and feel a little bit uncomfortable at first. This is a natural step to confront as many negative thoughts or fears, which are deeply rooted in our subconscious, sometimes stop many of us from going forward. You will have to break that vicious circle of passiveness and take charge of your destiny. Weight reductions or Life changes will only occur if you have decisively accepted to take charge and transform your life.

You can also apply that philosophy for work, inter family relationship or even to find love. Opportunity is endless, when you have decided that your life is in need of serious change. But I won't elaborate any further as so many books were written on self motivation but I do suggest that you read more in order to increase your positiveness.

Rewards

Section 11:

The rewards can be immense and quite uplifting, when you take the time to follow the above steps. You will feel in control of your life and demonstrated command of yourself within your society. The desires are yours to capture....

Like a cultural reader, immense in his knowledge of the world, you must decide to change your world. Yes there will be challenges or upsets, but you will have to drive your motivation to it's peek. If not, then your sacrifices would have been in vain, and you will be left to go back to your dull and none interesting life as an alternative. I don't want that to happen, so spark yourself and accept the challenge.

Another aspect of this program, is not to stop yourself from indulging in some fatty foods or treats once in a while, but merely to be reasonable. Those are small pleasures in life that we all appreciate, in moderation of course.

Example: After a successful week of applying this program, you could keep the weekend open for a meal at a restaurant or a popcorn or sweets to the movies. It could serve as an acknowledgment to your discipline weekly routine.

But as time goes by, you will easily adapt to your new found routine and find it more acceptable and pleasurable. The idea is to start and be consistent.

Bonus

Bonus:(Recipes, meal idea and calorie chart)

You will find enclosed a few recipes that you could easily use as a form of healthy nourishment.

Vegetarian Spaghetti:

Ingredients: Pasta, broccoli, carrots, onions, vegetable broth, sauce thickener.

First step: Cook a reasonable amount of pasta and put aside. In another dish pour in about four cups of water and bring to a boil. Incorporated the carrots and the vegetable(preferred) or chicken broth.

The proportion of broth within the suggested water ratios(2 tea spoons to a cup of water) will equal the manage portion of vegetables.

After about 7 minutes, you may add the broccoli and onions to cover the entire water surface. Don't worry the broccoli will become tender and blend in with the broth. You may also add mushrooms, peppers, or other vegetables to your dish.Bring to a boil five cups of water and incorporated about three table spoons of soy sauce. Pour in the carrots and wait for about 5 minutes before pouring in the remaining ingredients.

When your carrots are nice and tender and your bean sprouts are soft, remove all the water except for about ¼ of it, in order to finalized the side dish.

When all the vegetables are crisply cooked, taste the broth and simmer to taste. A dash of salt, or more syrup broth(don't add water or it will dilute the broth). Add your sauce thickener for consistency and serve over your pasta.

Vegetables Lite Gourmet:

Side portion for two.

Ingredients: Soy sauce, maple syrup, onions, carrots, mushrooms, bean sprouts.

Before starting cut three carrots, two small onions, ¼ cup of mushrooms and aside four cups of bean sprouts.

Pour the content in two separate bowls and add fresh soy sauce and maple syrup. Blend well within the vegetables and enjoy a most healthy side dish. The soy sauce and maple syrup may be added in tea spoons increment to reflect your personal taste.

Meal Idea: These are small personal suggestions that I was able to put together with the best lowest calorie intake.

Breakfast: Choose three only with side fruit dish.

Suggestion: Tea or coffee(no sugar or light substitute.)
          Pure juice or small glass of milk.

Homemade potato pancake	1 medium
Homemade French toast	1 only
Aunt Jemima Original pancakes	2 pancakes
Aunt Jemima Buttermilk pancakes	2 pancakes
Eggo Nutri-Grain Whole Wheat Waffles	1 waffle
Eggo Special K Fat Free Waffles	1 waffle
Egg white	1 large
Poached whole egg	1 large
Scrambles whole egg	1 large
Morningstar Farms breakfast Sausage Links	1 link
Alpha-Bits(cereals)	1 cup per cereal bowl

Cheerios (cereals)
Cookie Crisp
Corn Chex (cereals)
Corn Flakes(cereals)
Crispix
Froot Loops
Frosted Cheerios
Honey Nut Cheerios
Honeycomb
Kellogg's Pokemon
Kellogg's Special K with Red Berries
Lucky Charms
Multi-Grain Cheerios

Quaker Puffed Rice	
Quaker Puffed Wheat	
Special K	
Trix	
Wheaties	
Quaker Instant Oatmeal	1 pack
Quaker Instant lower Sugar Apples/Cinnamon	1 pack(oatmeal)
White Bread	2 slice
Reduced-calorie white bread	
Wonder White bread	
Whole Wheat bread	
Arnold Carb Counting Whole wheat bread	
Reduced-calorie wheat bread	
Pepperidge Farm Light Soft Wheat	
Pepperidge Farm Light 7 Grain	
Reduced-calorie Rye bread	
Breadsticks	1 only recommended
Diner roll	1 small
Supplements to Breakfast	
Sugar free jam	1 tbsp
Smucker's Sugar free jam(all flavors)	1 tbsp
Honey	1 tbsp
Molasses	1 tbsp
I can't believe it's not butter(fat free)	1 tbsp
I can't believe it's not butter(spray)	short spray
Margarine(stick)	1 tbsp
Fat Free American Cheese	1 slice best
Kraft Fat Free Singles(American)	1 slice
Philadelphia Fat Free Cream Cheese	2 tbsp acceptable
Kraft Fat Free Shredded Mozzarella.	25 cup(suggested)
Shredded Parmesan	1 tbsp
Kraft Parm Plus Parmesan with seasoning	2 tbsp
Velveeta Reduced fat	1 oz
Land O' Lakes Nonfat Sour cream	2 tbsp

Weight Watchers Light Sour Cream	2 tbsp
Coffee-Mate Nonfat Nondairy Creamer(Liquid)	1 tbsp
Coffee-Mate Nonfat Nondairy Creamer(powder)	1 tbsp
Nonfat(Skim) milk with Vitamin A	1 cup
Carnation low fat Evaporated milk	2 tbsp
Carnation Fat free Evaporated milk	2 tbsp
Westsoy Non Fat Soymilk Beverage	1 cup
Weight Watchers Chocolate Milk	1 serving

Diner/ supper

These meals should be supplemented with lots of fruits and vegetables. I have chosen a small selection accordingly to best calorie ratios. But I would like to stress that a homemade meal is always more preferable, then already made cook food or restaurants. This list should serve as a complement for individual with a highly time consuming routine. Use this list as a guideline within dining out or fast lunch routine.

Frozen Pizza: Bagel Bites 3 Cheese Bagel Pizza
Bagel Bites Cheese/sausage/Pepperoni
Little Caesar's Cheese only pizza
Little Caesar's Pepperoni pizza
Thin crust(12") Cheese
Thin crust(12") Pepperoni
Pizza Hut medium pan cheese pizza
Pizza Hut 14" large thin Chicken supreme
Pizza Hut 14" large thin Veggie lovers

Deli: Smoke Beef sausage
Kielbasa
Beef Bologna
Oscar Mayer Light Beef Bologna
Fat Free mesquite- flavored chicken breast
Oscar Mayer Oven Roasted Fat Free Chicken Breast

Jellied corned beef
Extra-lean slice ham
Oscar Mayer ham
Hormel Lite Spam
Chicken Liver Pate'
Turkey Salami
Turkey Breast(All highly recommended but fat free is better)
Hebrew National 97% Fat Free (wieners/hot dog)
Oscar Mayer Fat Free wiener
Homemade coleslaw
Chicken fried or cook but without the skin
McDonald's chicken nuggets (3 or less)

Note: Please take note that beef, ribs and steaks have a high density of calories, so the meat should be chosen with a lean context. Pork is a little bit more acceptable but should be carefully selected as fat free or with fat removed.

Fish offers the best beneficial value to the body within calories and Omega. I won't list them because mostly all of them are recommended. But do try to stay away from battered fish as a natural state is much more valuable. But for kids light weight battered fish could be an option in order to stimulate them to the taste.

For people on the go I would suggest the following alternative in frozen meals. I would also like to stress that a prepared meal at night before the next day work is preferable to the following options. Just look at the calorie box insert for references.

Weight Watchers Smart Ones Honey Dijon Chicken
Weight Watchers Smart Ones Shrimp Marinara
Amy's Organic Vegetable Shepherd's Pie

Soups: Campbell's Condensed Beef Consommé
Health Valley Fat Free Vegetable Broth
Progresso French Onion
Progresso Healthy Classic Chicken Noodle
Lipton Recipe Secrets Onion Soup mix
Lipton Cup-A-Soup Vegetable Soup Mix

Shoney's Tomato Soup with Vegetables

Dessert: Yogurt is always a recommended choice, but do try to compare the various blend for additional value . Values such as calcium or vitamins as a supplement, but do watch for the calories on the package.

For donuts, pastries, and candies they should be kept limited to one a day as a reward because of it's high density calorie content. Reward yourself as a source of pleasure on the weekend.

Calories Chart(Fruits)

This is a limited list that I have assembled for a glimpse of calorie value for some fruits. You may easily obtain such additional list within your library books or the Internet resource material.

Fruit	Cal.	Fruit	Fruit
Apple(medium)	65	Banana(medium)	90-100
Blackberries (½ cup)	36	Blueberries (½ cup)	41
Sweet Cherries (½ cup)	45	Cranberries (½ cup)	22
Grapefruit (1 medium)	82	Grapes (½ cup)	55
Lemon(1 medium)	24	Lime(one)	20
Kiwi(1 medium)	41	Mango(one)	135
Nectarine(one)	60	Cantaloupe(15% of one)	120 ave.
Honeydew melon(15%)	200 ave	Orange (1 medium)	70 ave.
Papaya(1 large)	148	Pear (1 medium)	95 ave.
Peaches(1 large)	61	Pineapple (½ cup) diced	37
Raspberries (½ cup)	32	Rhubarb (1 cup) diced	26
Strawberries (1 cup)	46	Watermelon (1 cup) diced	46

Calories Chart(Vegetables)

Vegetable	Cal.	Vegetable	Cal.
Asparagus (½ cup)	14	Beets (½ cup)	30 ave.
Broccoli (½ cup) chopped	16	Brussels sprout (½ cup)	19
Cabbage (½ cup) chopped	9 ave.	Carrots (1 large)	30
Cauliflower (½ cup)	12	Celery (½ cup) chopped	7
Cucumber (1 large)	36 ave.	Eggplant (½ cup) cubes	10
Garlic(2 cloves)	8 ave.	Lettuce (½ cup) shredded	4
Romaine lettuce (½ cup)	4	Mushrooms (½ cup)	8 ave.
Onions (½ cup) chopped	34	Green pepper(1 large)	33
Red pepper(1 medium)	35	Radish(10)	10
Spinach (½ cup)	4 ave.	Turnips (1 medium)	40
Tomatoes(1 medium)	22	Zucchini (1 medium)	40

The above products were calculated on an average scale and are in their raw state. I listed the most popular products, by more are available upon research within the net, local libraries or governmental health guidelines resource materials.

Conclusion

I hope that all of these small hints have been beneficial to you, and that you have decided to follow all of its main points. I hope that you will gracefully apply them as my main focus is to share a program that has successfully work for me. In the last few months I was inspired, and motivated by so much interesting changes in my life. I went from and obese person to a more slimmer and normal weight individual. My life was also totally transform with a desire for changes and new direction. I became less passive, and became aware of my new found energy. I'm also aware that we all have our own limitations that we can absorb in a program, but this will definitely be a good start. Even if you only change half of your life due to this information package well at least you still have reaped a reward.

My intention was merely to inform you of a most valuable alternative to all those exuberant and expensive weight reduction programs. They make you pay for their services, meal programs, pills, books, dvd etc.... The only thing that is required is common sense and sound eating practices. The secret is in controlling the calories intake that goes into your body pertaining to the ones that is required. A little bit of exercise(walking etc..)along with a balance diet and a new mental attitude would be the proven solution to your success. GOOD LUCK

Disclosure

Like everything pertaining to the general welfare of the population, I must acknowledge that I am not a doctor or dietitian. So if in doubt please refer to your health specialist. My facts are base from my personal weight reduction experience along with various sources research material. I'm also aware that weight reductions loss is totally subject to time and effort apply by an individual and that it is not a specific science. So without due hesitation, I wish to congratulated you into taking a fresh new step into and overall life changing experience. Enjoy your new found journey in the world of self control.

Yvan F. Leger

Biography

Yvan Leger was born and raise in Cornwall, Ontario, Canada. He attended St.Gabriel elementary School, Jean XX111 and LaCitadelle High School. He also serve as a Captain within the military and eventually became the Commanding Officer of 325 Air cadet Squadron. He work diligently within the family business and eventually founded Y.F.Leger Creational Wear Canada(Ltd) in 1994. He created the line of clothes Sweet and Pretty and Baby Cuddle. In 2010 he became a fashion designer under it's exclusive line of products. At his own time Yvan Leger write books, entertained himself in music and his currently in the stage of an invention that his currently under review for the automobile industry.